VIRIN GOMBER

Trivia For Seniors

200 Multiple-Choice Nostalgic Quiz Questions and Brain Activity to Boost Your Memory (Large Print)

First edition

This book was professionally typeset on Reedsy.
Find out more at reedsy.com

"Life can only be understood backwards; but it must be lived forwards."

- SØREN KIERKEGAARD

Contents

1

INTRODUCTION

This Trivia book is a tailored journey into the past, aimed at providing you with a stimulating and enjoyable way to engage your mind.

It has been created to offer an engaging, fun, and mentally stimulating experience for all adults, especially seniors. By diving into the rich tapestry of the past decades, from the Fifties to the Nineties, this book aims to evoke memories, prompt discussions, and keep your mind sharp.

Each chapter in this book focuses on a different decade and is packed with questions that cover various aspects of that era, including music, movies, history, and culture. The questions are formatted in a multiple-choice style for ease of use and accessibility, and the large print format ensures it's easy on your eyes.

Trivia quizzes have been shown to help maintain cognitive function, boost memory, and encourage learning. They're a fun way to challenge yourself and learn new things, keeping your brain active and engaged.

As you go through this book, remember that the goal isn't just to answer the questions correctly. It's about the experience – the thinking, the reminiscing, and the discussions that each question brings about.

Getting the Most Out of Your Trivia Book

To truly benefit from "Trivia For Seniors," consider the following tips:

- **Take Your Time:** There's no rush to complete the book. Enjoy each question, ponder over the choices, and relish the memories or knowledge each one brings.
- **Make It Social:** This book can be an excellent tool for interaction with friends, family, or fellow seniors. Use it as a conversation starter or as a fun group activity.
- **Embrace Learning:** If you encounter a question about something unfamiliar, take it as an opportunity to learn something new.
- **Reminisce and Share Stories:** Let the questions trigger your memories. Share your stories and experiences related to the topics in the book.
- **Regular Engagement:** Try to engage with the book regularly. Consistent mental stimulation is vital to keeping your brain sharp.
- **Enjoy the Journey:** Above all, have fun! This book is about enjoying the journey through the past, embracing nostalgia, and celebrating a lifetime of experiences.

As we begin with "The Fifties," prepare to be transported to a time of rock 'n' roll, significant cultural shifts, and historical milestones. Each chapter after that will take you through a successive decade, enriching your knowledge and triggering fond memories.

2

THE FIFTIES

Welcome to the fabulous 1950s – a decade known for its cultural revolutions, historical milestones, and the birth of iconic pop culture moments. Dive into a collection of 40 handpicked trivia questions that capture the essence of the 1950s.

Trivia Questions from the 50s

1. Who was the President of the United States at the start of the 1950s?
   a. Harry S. Truman
   b. Dwight D. Eisenhower
   c. Franklin D. Roosevelt
   d. John F. Kennedy

2. What was the first animated feature film released by Disney in the 1950s?
   a. Cinderella
   b. Alice in Wonderland
   c. Peter Pan

    d. Sleeping Beauty

2. In 1951, which country's troops entered the Korean War to assist North Korea?

    a. Soviet Union

    b. China

    c. Japan

    d. Vietnam

4. Which iconic music genre is said to have been born in the 1950s?

    a. Jazz

    b. Rock 'n' Roll

    c. R&B

    d. Hip Hop

5. What was the name of the first artificial Earth satellite, launched in 1957?

    a. Explorer 1

    b. Sputnik 1

    c. Vanguard 1

    d. Apollo 11

6. Who wrote the influential novel '1984', published in 1949 but gaining popularity in the 1950s?

    a. George Orwell

    b. Aldous Huxley

    c. Ray Bradbury

    d. J.D. Salinger

7. In 1954, Roger Bannister became the first person to run a mile in under how many minutes?

    a. 3 minutes

    b. 4 minutes

   c. 5 minutes
   d. 6 minutes

8. Which movie starring Marlon Brando became a cultural phenomenon in 1953?

   a. On the Waterfront
   b. A Streetcar Named Desire
   c. The Wild One
   d. Rebel Without a Cause

9. Which year did the iconic Disneyland Park open during the 1950s?

   a. 1950
   b. 1952
   c. 1955
   d. 1958

10. In 1959, Fidel Castro came to power in which country?

   a. Mexico
   b. Brazil
   c. Cuba
   d. Venezuela

11. Which famous musician died in a plane crash on February 3, 1959, known as 'The Day the Music Died'?

   a. Elvis Presley
   b. Buddy Holly
   c. Chuck Berry
   d. Johnny Cash

12. Which actress starred in 'I Love Lucy,' a popular TV show from the 1950s?

   a. Lucille Ball
   b. Marilyn Monroe

   c. Audrey Hepburn

   d. Elizabeth Taylor

13. What was the first color television show to be broadcast in the 1950s?

   a. The Ed Sullivan Show

   b. The Adventures of Ozzie and Harriet

   c. I Love Lucy

   d. Bonanza

14. Who was the author of 'The Catcher in the Rye,' a novel that became immensely popular among teenagers in the 1950s?

   a. Ernest Hemingway

   b. J.D. Salinger

   c. F. Scott Fitzgerald

   d. William Faulkner

15. In 1954, the U.S. Supreme Court made a landmark decision in which case, declaring racial segregation in public schools unconstitutional?

   a. Plessy v. Ferguson

   b. Brown v. Board of Education

   c. Roe v. Wade

   d. Marbury v. Madison

16. Which popular board game, still played today, was first published by Parker Brothers in the 1950s?

   a. Risk

   b. Scrabble

   c. Monopoly

   d. Clue

17. What was the predominant style of music among teenagers in the 1950s?

a. Jazz

b. Rock 'n' Roll

c. Blues

d. Country

18. In 1953, who became the first woman to be crowned Queen of the United Kingdom in the 20th century?

a. Queen Elizabeth II

b. Queen Mary II

c. Queen Victoria

d. Queen Anne

19. The first successful vaccine for which disease was developed in 1955?

a. Polio

b. Measles

c. Smallpox

d. Tuberculosis

20. Which iconic film star married Joe DiMaggio in 1954?

a. Audrey Hepburn

b. Elizabeth Taylor

c. Marilyn Monroe

d. Grace Kelly

21. What was the famous catchphrase of comedian Jerry Lewis during the 1950s?

a. "Nice lady!"

b. "Hey, Abbott!"

c. "That's all folks!"

d. "You bet your life!"

22. Who broke the color barrier in Major League Baseball in 1947 and

became an icon in the 1950s?

a. Hank Aaron

b. Willie Mays

c. Jackie Robinson

d. Satchel Paige

23. Which author wrote the novel 'Lolita,' which stirred much controversy upon its release?

a. Vladimir Nabokov

b. Ernest Hemingway

c. J.D. Salinger

d. John Steinbeck

24. Which car became synonymous with the 1950s and is often associated with the era's culture?

a. Ford Mustang

b. Chevrolet Bel Air

c. Volkswagen Beetle

d. Cadillac Eldorado

25. What historic event took place on October 4, 1957, marking the beginning of the Space Age?

a. The first man walked on the moon.

b. The first artificial satellite, Sputnik, was launched.

c. The first human traveled into space.

d. The Hubble Space Telescope was launched.

26. What popular children's toy, which can 'walk' downstairs, was invented in the 1950s?

a. Hula Hoop

b. Slinky

c. Barbie Doll

d. Mr. Potato Head

27. Which Alfred Hitchcock film, released in 1954, became a classic thriller?

a. Psycho

b. Vertigo

c. Rear Window

d. North by Northwest

28. In 1958, NASA was established in response to the space achievements of which country?

a. Germany

b. Russia

c. Japan

d. China

29. Which famous musical featuring rival gangs in New York City debuted on Broadway in 1957?

a. Oklahoma!

b. The Sound of Music

c. West Side Story

d. My Fair Lady

30. In 1956, who released the hit song 'Heartbreak Hotel'?

a. Frank Sinatra

b. Elvis Presley

c. Buddy Holly

d. Chuck Berry

31. Which groundbreaking sitcom premiered in 1951 featuring a mixed-race couple?

a. The Honeymooners

b. I Love Lucy

c. Leave it to Beaver

d. The Dick Van Dyke Show

32. What was the first commercial jet airliner introduced in the 1950s?
   a. Boeing 707
   b. Douglas DC-8
   c. De Havilland Comet
   d. Lockheed Constellation

33. In 1952, which major city was enveloped by the Great Smog, leading to significant changes in environmental policies?
   a. New York
   b. London
   c. Paris
   d. Tokyo

34. Who wrote the science fiction classic 'Fahrenheit 451', published in 1953?
   a. Isaac Asimov
   b. Arthur C. Clarke
   c. Ray Bradbury
   d. Philip K. Dick

35. Which iconic film, released in 1957, stars Henry Fonda and is set in a jury deliberation room?
   a. Vertigo
   b. 12 Angry Men
   c. Rebel Without a Cause
   d. On the Waterfront

36. What popular dance style originated in the 1950s?
   a. The Twist
   b. The Jitterbug
   c. The Cha-Cha
   d. Rock 'n' Roll

37. In 1954, which Asian country was divided at the 17th parallel after the Indochina War?
   a. Korea
   b. Vietnam
   c. China
   d. Japan

38. Which iconic 1950s TV show was hosted by Rod Serling?
   a. The Twilight Zone
   b. Alfred Hitchcock Presents
   c. The Outer Limits
   d. Dragnet

39. Who wrote 'The Old Man and the Sea', which won the Nobel Prize in Literature in 1954?
   a. Ernest Hemingway
   b. William Faulkner
   c. John Steinbeck
   d. F. Scott Fitzgerald

40. What was the major political event in 1956 involving Egypt and the control of the Suez Canal?
   a. The Suez Crisis
   b. The Six-Day War
   c. The Yom Kippur War
   d. The Arab-Israeli War

One Special Memory from the 50s

"The Launch of Sputnik 1 - The event on October 4, 1957, that marked the beginning of the space age and symbolized the height of the Cold War space race."

As we conclude this chapter on the 1950s, it's not just a farewell to a decade but an appreciation of a time that set many wheels in motion, shaping the world as we know it today. The next chapter will usher us into the Swinging Sixties, a decade of radical change and vibrant expression.

3

THE SIXTIES

The 1960s was a decade of profound change and remarkable happenings, touching every aspect of human life. From the heights of space exploration with the Apollo moon landing to the depths of social upheaval with the Civil Rights Movement, the Sixties were a time of both achievements and challenges.

Trivia Questions from the 60s

1. Who became the first man to walk on the moon in 1969?
   a. Neil Armstrong
   b. Buzz Aldrin
   c. John Glenn
   d. Yuri Gagarin

2. Which band released the hit album 'Sgt. Pepper's Lonely Hearts Club Band' in 1967?
   a. The Beatles
   b. The Rolling Stones
   c. The Beach Boys

d. The Who

3. In 1963, who delivered the famous 'I Have a Dream' speech?
   a. Malcolm X
   b. Martin Luther King Jr.
   c. John F. Kennedy
   d. Nelson Mandela

4. Which movie featuring the character of Mrs. Robinson was a hit in 1967?
   a. Breakfast at Tiffany's
   b. The Graduate
   c. Bonnie and Clyde
   d. West Side Story

5. What was the major global event from 1962 known as the closest the Cold War came to escalating into full-scale nuclear war?
   a. The Berlin Crisis
   b. The Cuban Missile Crisis
   c. The Korean War
   d. The Vietnam War

6. Which famous music festival took place in 1969, symbolizing the peak of the hippie movement?
   a. Monterey Pop Festival
   b. Woodstock
   c. Isle of Wight Festival
   d. Altamont Free Concert

7. Who assassinated U.S. President John F. Kennedy in 1963?
   a. Lee Harvey Oswald
   b. Sirhan Sirhan
   c. James Earl Ray

d. Mark David Chapman

8. Which best-selling book by Harper Lee, published in 1960, became an instant classic?
   a. To Kill a Mockingbird
   b. Catch-22
   c. Brave New World
   d. Lord of the Flies

9. In 1961, which astronaut became the first American to travel into space?
   a. John Glenn
   b. Neil Armstrong
   c. Alan Shepard
   d. Gus Grissom

10. Which iconic car, known for its role in the 1960s counterculture movement, was introduced by Volkswagen in the US?
   a. The Beetle
   b. The Minibus
   c. The Microbus
   d. The Karmann Ghia

11. Which amendment to the U.S. Constitution, ratified in 1964, outlawed poll taxes?
   a. 22nd Amendment
   b. 23rd Amendment
   c. 24th Amendment
   d. 25th Amendment

12. Who was the influential British Prime Minister during much of the 1960s?
   a. Winston Churchill

b. Harold Wilson

c. Margaret Thatcher

d. Anthony Eden

13. What was the name of the first successful American sitcom to feature a predominantly African American cast?

a. The Jeffersons

b. Good Times

c. Julia

d. I Spy

14. In 1967, which territory did Israel capture during the Six-Day War?

a. Gaza Strip

b. Golan Heights

c. West Bank

d. All of the above

15. Who wrote the classic 1961 novel 'Catch-22'?

a. Joseph Heller

b. Kurt Vonnegut

c. J.D. Salinger

d. Harper Lee

16. Which contraceptive was first approved by the FDA in 1960?

a. The birth control pill

b. IUD

c. Condom

d. Diaphragm

17. Which 1969 film starring Paul Newman and Robert Redford was a major hit and classic?

a. The Sting

b. Cool Hand Luke

   c. Butch Cassidy and the Sundance Kid

   d. The Hustler

18. In 1960, which country gained independence from Belgium, leading to significant political changes in Africa?

   a. Rwanda

   b. The Congo

   c. Uganda

   d. Kenya

19. What was the major environmental disaster that struck the United Kingdom in 1966, known as the Aberfan disaster?

   a. A nuclear meltdown

   b. A coal mine collapse

   c. A landslide

   d. An oil spill

20. Who was the first African American Supreme Court Justice, appointed in 1967?

   a. Clarence Thomas

   b. Thurgood Marshall

   c. Colin Powell

   d. Frederick Douglass

21. Which popular 1960s TV show featured a group of castaways stranded on an uncharted island?

   a. The Twilight Zone

   b. Gilligan's Island

   c. Lost in Space

   d. Star Trek

22. Which album by The Beach Boys, released in 1966, is often considered one of the greatest in rock music history?

a. Pet Sounds
b. Surf's Up
c. Smile
d. Sunflower

23. What was the landmark event of the Civil Rights Movement that took place in August 1963?

a. The Montgomery Bus Boycott
b. The March on Washington
c. The Birmingham Campaign
d. The Freedom Rides

24. In which year did the Vietnam War officially begin?

a. 1960
b. 1962
c. 1964
d. 1965

25. Which iconic 1960s film is known for its shower scene, directed by Alfred Hitchcock?

a. Vertigo
b. Psycho
c. North by Northwest
d. The Birds

26. Which famous civil rights activist was assassinated in 1968?

a. Malcolm X
b. Martin Luther King Jr.
c. Medgar Evers
d. Fred Hampton

27. What was the best-selling car model in the 1960s, symbolizing the era's automotive culture?

a. Ford Mustang

b. Chevrolet Impala

c. Volkswagen Beetle

d. Pontiac GTO

28. Who was the first woman to travel into space in 1963?

a. Sally Ride

b. Valentina Tereshkova

c. Mae Jemison

d. Eileen Collins

29. Which 1968 movie by Stanley Kubrick is known for its groundbreaking visuals and deep philosophical themes?

a. Dr. Strangelove

b. A Clockwork Orange

c. 2001: A Space Odyssey

d. Full Metal Jacket

30. Which amendment to the U.S. Constitution, passed in 1961, allowed residents of Washington D.C. to vote in presidential elections?

a. 22nd Amendment

b. 23rd Amendment

c. 24th Amendment

d. 25th Amendment

31. In 1964, which group arrived in the U.S. and appeared on 'The Ed Sullivan Show,' marking the start of the British Invasion?

a. The Beatles

b. The Rolling Stones

c. The Who

d. The Kinks

32. What was the controversial war strategy used by the U.S. in Vietnam,

involving extensive aerial bombing?
   a. Napalm strikes
   b. Guerrilla warfare
   c. Operation Rolling Thunder
   d. Search and destroy missions

33.   Which influential book by Rachel Carson, published in 1962, sparked the modern environmental movement?
   a. The Sea Around Us
   b. Silent Spring
   c. The Sense of Wonder
   d. The Edge of the Sea

34. Who was the heavyweight boxing champion of the world for most of the 1960s?
   a. Muhammad Ali
   b. Joe Frazier
   c. Sonny Liston
   d. George Foreman

35. Which 1961 movie musical, starring Natalie Wood, is a retelling of Romeo and Juliet set in New York City?
   a. My Fair Lady
   b. West Side Story
   c. The Sound of Music
   d. Grease

36. In 1960, which African country became the first to gain independence from British rule?
   a. Kenya
   b. Nigeria
   c. Ghana
   d. South Africa

37. What major U.S. event happened in 1969 that is often cited as the end of the innocence of the 1960s?
   a. The Moon Landing
   b. Woodstock
   c. The Manson Family murders
   d. The assassination of Robert F. Kennedy

38. Who was the U.S. President at the end of the 1960s?
   a. John F. Kennedy
   b. Lyndon B. Johnson
   c. Richard Nixon
   d. Dwight D. Eisenhower

39. Which event marked the official start of the feminist movement in the 1960s?
   a. The publication of "The Feminine Mystique"
   b. The founding of NOW (National Organization for Women)
   c. The Women's Strike for Equality
   d. The passing of the Equal Pay Act

40. Which iconic music event was held in San Francisco's Golden Gate Park in 1967?
   a. The Monterey Pop Festival
   b. The Human Be-In
   c. Woodstock
   d. Altamont Free Concert

One Special Memory from the 60s

"Apollo 11 Moon Landing - The monumental event on July 20, 1969, when Neil Armstrong and Buzz Aldrin became the first humans to step on the moon, marking a pinnacle in space exploration."

As we leave behind the tumultuous yet groundbreaking Sixties, we transition into the Seventies - a decade known for its unique blend of cultural, political, and technological developments.

4

THE SEVENTIES

The 1970s, often remembered for its distinctive style and transformative events, was a decade marked by its unique fashion, influential music, and significant socio-political movements. It also saw the world navigating through the complexities of the Cold War, the energy crisis, and the quest for civil rights and environmental awareness.

Trivia Questions from the 70s

1. Who was the U.S. President who resigned in 1974 due to the Watergate scandal?
   a. Richard Nixon
   b. Gerald Ford
   c. Jimmy Carter
   d. Lyndon B. Johnson

2. Which blockbuster movie, directed by Steven Spielberg, was released in 1975 and became a huge hit?
   a. Star Wars
   b. Jaws

   c. Close Encounters of the Third Kind

   d. Rocky

3. What was the popular dance style that originated in the 1970s and was associated with the disco movement?

   a. The Twist

   b. Breakdancing

   c. The Hustle

   d. The Moonwalk

4. Which technology was introduced by Sony in 1979, revolutionizing personal music listening?

   a. The CD Player

   b. The Walkman

   c. The Boombox

   d. The MP3 Player

5. Who became the first female Prime Minister of the United Kingdom in 1979?

   a. Indira Gandhi

   b. Golda Meir

   c. Margaret Thatcher

   d. Angela Merkel

6. The 1970s saw the end of the Vietnam War. In which year did U.S. troops officially withdraw?

   a. 1973

   b. 1975

   c. 1970

   d. 1977

7. Which iconic 1977 film began the 'Star Wars' saga, directed by George Lucas?

a. Star Wars: A New Hope

b. Star Wars: The Empire Strikes Back

c. Star Wars: Return of the Jedi

d. Star Wars: The Phantom Menace

8. What was the name of the space station that crashed back to Earth in 1979?

a. Mir

b. Salyut 1

c. Skylab

d. International Space Station

9. Which music genre, characterized by a fast tempo and aggressive lyrics, emerged in the 1970s?

a. Disco

b. Punk Rock

c. Heavy Metal

d. Reggae

10. In 1971, which country changed its name from East Pakistan to its current name?

a. Bangladesh

b. Myanmar

c. Sri Lanka

d. Nepal

11. Which environmental celebration was first observed on April 22, 1970?

a. Earth Hour

b. Earth Day

c. World Environment Day

d. Arbor Day

12. Which groundbreaking arcade video game, released in 1978, became a cultural phenomenon?

    a. Space Invaders

    b. Pong

    c. Pac-Man

    d. Asteroids

13. In 1972, which U.S. President made a historic visit to China, beginning the process of normalizing relations between the two countries?

    a. Richard Nixon

    b. Jimmy Carter

    c. Gerald Ford

    d. Lyndon B. Johnson

14. Who was the notorious serial killer arrested in the 1970s, known for his charismatic personality and heinous crimes?

    a. Charles Manson

    b. Ted Bundy

    c. John Wayne Gacy

    d. Jeffrey Dahmer

15. Which legendary rock and roll musician, known as 'The King,' died in 1977?

    a. Elvis Presley

    b. John Lennon

    c. Jimi Hendrix

    d. Freddie Mercury

16. What was the name of the scandal involving illegal wiretapping that led to President Nixon's resignation?

    a. Iran-Contra Affair

    b. Teapot Dome Scandal

    c. Watergate Scandal

    d. Whitewater Scandal

17. Which landmark U.S. Supreme Court case in 1973 legalized abortion?

    a. Brown v. Board of Education

    b. Roe v. Wade

    c. Plessy v. Ferguson

    d. Miranda v. Arizona

18. Who won the heavyweight boxing match known as 'The Rumble in the Jungle' in 1974?

    a. George Foreman

    b. Muhammad Ali

    c. Joe Frazier

    d. Ken Norton

19. Which 1976 film about a boxing underdog won the Academy Award for Best Picture?

    a. Rocky

    b. Raging Bull

    c. The Godfather

    d. Taxi Driver

20. In 1978, which country became the first to legalize same-sex sexual relations?

    a. Sweden

    b. Netherlands

    c. Canada

    d. France

21. What famous rock band broke up in 1970, leading to successful solo careers for its members?

a. The Beatles
b. The Rolling Stones
c. Led Zeppelin
d. Pink Floyd

22. Which car company introduced the iconic Golf model in 1974?
a. Ford
b. Toyota
c. Volkswagen
d. Honda

23. What was the pivotal environmental law passed in the U.S. in 1970 that created the Environmental Protection Agency (EPA)?
a. Clean Air Act
b. National Environmental Policy Act
c. Clean Water Act
d. Endangered Species Act

24. In 1976, Apple Inc. was founded by Steve Jobs, Steve Wozniak, and which other individual?
a. Bill Gates
b. Ronald Wayne
c. Paul Allen
d. Michael Dell

25. Which hit TV show from the 1970s, set during the Korean War, featured the staff of a mobile army surgical hospital?
a. MASH
b. The Waltons
c. All in the Family
d. Happy Days

26. Which 1973 album by Pink Floyd is known for its iconic prism

cover art and is one of the best-selling albums of all time?
   a. Animals
   b. The Dark Side of the Moon
   c. Wish You Were Here
   d. The Wall

27. Who became the first female Secretary of State in the United States in 1977?
   a. Madeleine Albright
   b. Condoleezza Rice
   c. Hillary Clinton
   d. Jean Kirkpatrick

28. Which event, occurring in 1979, led to a prolonged hostage crisis involving American embassy staff in Iran?
   a. The Gulf War
   b. The Iran-Iraq War
   c. The Iranian Revolution
   d. Operation Eagle Claw

29. In 1979, which nuclear power plant in the United States suffered a partial meltdown, raising concerns about nuclear energy safety?
   a. Three Mile Island
   b. Chernobyl
   c. Fukushima
   d. Hanford Site

30. Which popular arcade game, released in 1978, is known for its simple yet addictive gameplay involving defending against rows of alien invaders?
   a. Space Invaders
   b. Asteroids
   c. Pac-Man

d. Pong

31. What was the name of the peace treaty signed between Israel and Egypt in 1979, facilitated by U.S. President Jimmy Carter?
a. The Oslo Accords
b. The Camp David Accords
c. The Geneva Accords
d. The Treaty of Versailles

32. In 1975, Microsoft was founded by Bill Gates and which other individual?
a. Steve Jobs
b. Paul Allen
c. Larry Ellison
d. Mark Zuckerberg

33. Which 1971 film, directed by Stanley Kubrick, is known for its dystopian themes and controversial subject matter?
a. 2001: A Space Odyssey
b. A Clockwork Orange
c. The Shining
d. Full Metal Jacket

34. In 1971, which country was the first to grant women the right to vote in national elections?
a. Switzerland
b. United States
c. Sweden
d. Canada

35. Which famous martial artist and actor starred in the 1973 film 'Enter the Dragon'?
a. Bruce Lee

b. Jackie Chan

c. Chuck Norris

d. Jet Li

36. What iconic rock festival was held in New York in 1969 and is often associated with the counterculture of the 1970s?

a. Woodstock

b. Monterey Pop Festival

c. Altamont Free Concert

d. Isle of Wight Festival

37. Which famous American director released the groundbreaking horror film 'The Exorcist' in 1973?

a. Steven Spielberg

b. George Lucas

c. William Friedkin

d. Martin Scorsese

38. What was the name of the first video game console released by Atari in 1977?

a. Atari 2600

b. Magnavox Odyssey

c. Nintendo Entertainment System

d. Sega Genesis

39. Which U.S. Supreme Court case in 1978 upheld the use of affirmative action in college admissions?

a. Brown v. Board of Education

b. Regents of the University of California v. Bakke

c. Roe v. Wade

d. Miranda v. Arizona

40. In 1971, John Lennon released which famous song as a single, which

has since become an anthem for peace?

    a. "Imagine"
    b. "Let It Be"
    c. "Yesterday"
    d. "Hey Jude"

One Special Memory from the 70s

"The First Test-Tube Baby - In 1978, Louise Brown became the world's first baby to be conceived via in vitro fertilization (IVF), marking a milestone in reproductive technology."

As we leave the dynamic and diverse Seventies, we move into the Eighties - a decade known for its cultural vibrancy, technological leaps, and global events that continued to shape the modern era.

5

THE EIGHTIES

The 1980s was a dynamic decade marked by vivid cultural changes, technological innovation, and pivotal global events. From the rise of digital technology and video games to the fall of the Berlin Wall, the Eighties were characterized by rapid advancements and significant political shifts.

Trivia Questions from the 80s

1. Who was the U.S. President throughout most of the 1980s?
   a. Ronald Reagan
   b. Jimmy Carter
   c. George H.W. Bush
   d. Bill Clinton

2. Which 1985 science fiction film features a high school student who travels back in time in a DeLorean car?
   a. Blade Runner
   b. The Terminator
   c. Back to the Future

d. E.T. the Extra-Terrestrial

3. What was the name of the nuclear power plant in Ukraine that suffered a catastrophic meltdown in 1986?
a. Three Mile Island
b. Fukushima Daiichi
c. Chernobyl
d. Kursk

4. Which artist released the hit album 'Thriller' in 1982, becoming the best-selling album of all time?
a. Michael Jackson
b. Madonna
c. Prince
d. Whitney Houston

5. In 1983, which technology was introduced that revolutionized home entertainment by allowing people to record and play videos?
a. DVD player
b. Blu-ray
c. VCR
d. LaserDisc

6. Which space shuttle tragically exploded shortly after launch in 1986?
a. Challenger
b. Discovery
c. Atlantis
d. Endeavour

7. Who was the British Prime Minister throughout most of the 1980s?
a. Margaret Thatcher
b. John Major
c. Tony Blair

    d. Winston Churchill

8. Which video game featuring a plumber who rescues Princess Peach became a cultural icon in the 1980s?
    a. Sonic the Hedgehog
    b. Super Mario Bros.
    c. Pac-Man
    d. Space Invaders

9. What was the name of the first woman appointed to the U.S. Supreme Court in 1981?
    a. Ruth Bader Ginsburg
    b. Sandra Day O'Connor
    c. Elena Kagan
    d. Sonia Sotomayor

10. Which disease was identified in the early 1980s, leading to a major global health crisis?
    a. Ebola
    b. SARS
    c. HIV/AIDS
    d. H1N1 Influenza

11. Which popular TV show featuring a group of friends in New York debuted in 1989?
    a. Friends
    b. Seinfeld
    c. Cheers
    d. Frasier

12. In 1981, MTV was launched, revolutionizing the music industry. What was the first music video played on MTV?
    a. "Thriller" by Michael Jackson

b. "Like a Virgin" by Madonna

c. "Video Killed the Radio Star" by The Buggles

d. "Money for Nothing" by Dire Straits

13. Which iconic 1980s film featured a time-traveling car and a flux capacitor?

a. Blade Runner

b. Tron

c. Back to the Future

d. The Terminator

14. Who was the first female artist inducted into the Rock and Roll Hall of Fame in 1988?

a. Aretha Franklin

b. Tina Turner

c. Janis Joplin

d. Madonna

15. In 1983, Sally Ride became the first American woman to do what?

a. Win a Nobel Prize

b. Become a Supreme Court Justice

c. Travel into space

d. Run for President

16. Which action movie, released in 1988, became a Christmas classic starring Bruce Willis?

a. Die Hard

b. Lethal Weapon

c. Predator

d. Rambo

17. What was the bestselling video game console of the 1980s?

a. Sega Genesis

b. Nintendo Entertainment System

c. Atari 2600

d. Commodore 64

18. The 1987 treaty known as the INF Treaty was signed between the United States and which other country?

a. China

b. Soviet Union

c. Germany

d. United Kingdom

19. Which 1980s TV series starred Don Johnson and Philip Michael Thomas as two Miami detectives?

a. Miami Vice

b. Magnum P.I.

c. Hill Street Blues

d. The A-Team

20.   What was the environmental disaster that occurred in 1989 involving a massive oil spill off the coast of Alaska?

a. Deepwater Horizon oil spill

b. Exxon Valdez oil spill

c. BP oil spill

d. Amoco Cadiz oil spill

21. Which fitness program, led by Jane Fonda, became a craze in the 1980s?

a. Zumba

b. Pilates

c. Aerobics

d. Yoga

22. Which novel by Margaret Atwood, published in 1985, depicts a

dystopian future and later became a successful TV series?
    a. The Handmaid's Tale
    b. Cat's Eye
    c. Alias Grace
    d. The Blind Assassin

23. What was the name of the popular toy robot, introduced in 1982, that could be programmed to carry small objects and perform tasks?
    a. Robosapien
    b. Omnibot
    c. AIBO
    d. R.O.B.

24. Which band, known for their flamboyant lead singer, released the iconic album 'Thriller' in 1982?
    a. Queen
    b. Michael Jackson
    c. U2
    d. Guns N' Roses

25. Which 1986 movie, starring Tom Cruise as a fighter pilot, became a symbol of 80s action cinema?
    a. Top Gun
    b. Iron Eagle
    c. The Right Stuff
    d. Red Dawn

26. In 1985, which historic Live Aid concerts were held to raise funds for famine relief in Ethiopia?
    a. Woodstock
    b. Live Aid
    c. Farm Aid
    d. Sun City

27. What was the first feature-length computer-animated movie released by Pixar in 1989?

a. Toy Story

b. The Little Mermaid

c. Tron

d. Luxo Jr.

28. Which tennis player dominated the sport in the 1980s with multiple Grand Slam victories?

a. Andre Agassi

b. Pete Sampras

c. John McEnroe

d. Bjorn Borg

29. In 1989, the first GPS satellite was launched by which country?

a. United States

b. Soviet Union

c. Japan

d. China

30. Which iconic music video by Michael Jackson featuring zombie dancers was released in 1983 and became a massive hit?

a. Beat It

b. Thriller

c. Bad

d. Billie Jean

31. Who was the influential leader of the Soviet Union during the latter half of the 1980s, known for his policies of Glasnost and Perestroika?

a. Leonid Brezhnev

b. Mikhail Gorbachev

c. Boris Yeltsin

d. Vladimir Putin

32. Which iconic action movie character, portrayed by Sylvester Stallone, first appeared in the 1982 film 'First Blood'?
   a. Rocky Balboa
   b. John Rambo
   c. The Terminator
   d. Indiana Jones

33. In 1983, which TV miniseries about an alien invasion became one of the most-watched programs of the year?
   a. Battlestar Galactica
   b. Star Trek: The Next Generation
   c. V
   d. Quantum Leap

34. Which 1980s video game featuring a yellow character eating dots in a maze while evading ghosts became a cultural icon?
   a. Space Invaders
   b. Donkey Kong
   c. Pac-Man
   d. Tetris

35. What was the best-selling book of the 1980s, written by Tom Wolfe and known for its portrayal of New York City life?
   a. The Bonfire of the Vanities
   b. The Color Purple
   c. Beloved
   d. Bright Lights, Big City

36. Which famous artist's painting, 'Irises,' set a record for the highest price ever paid for an artwork at auction in 1987?
   a. Vincent van Gogh
   b. Pablo Picasso
   c. Claude Monet

d. Andy Warhol

37. Which major environmental disaster, involving the release of a toxic gas, occurred in Bhopal, India in 1984?
   a. Chernobyl disaster
   b. Bhopal gas tragedy
   c. Exxon Valdez oil spill
   d. Seveso disaster

38. In 1989, which computer scientist invented the World Wide Web?
   a. Steve Jobs
   b. Bill Gates
   c. Tim Berners-Lee
   d. Mark Zuckerberg

39. Which famous horror author published 'It,' a best-selling novel, in 1986?
   a. Stephen King
   b. Dean Koontz
   c. Anne Rice
   d. Clive Barker

40. Who was the first African American Miss America crowned in 1983?
   a. Halle Berry
   b. Oprah Winfrey
   c. Vanessa Williams
   d. Tyra Banks

One Special Memory from the 80s

"The Fall of the Berlin Wall - In 1989, this symbol of the Cold War was brought down, signifying the end of the division between East and West Germany and a major step towards the end of the Cold War."

Leaving the colorful and eventful Eighties behind, we transition to the Nineties. This decade, known for its technological advancements and cultural shifts, set the stage for the new millennium.

6

THE NINETIES

The 1990s was a decade of significant global transformations and cultural milestones. This was a period marked by the end of the Cold War, the rise of the Internet, and the emergence of a new pop culture landscape.

Trivia Questions from the 90s

1. Who was elected as President of the United States in 1992, ending 12 years of Republican presidency?
   a. George H.W. Bush
   b. Bill Clinton
   c. Al Gore
   d. George W. Bush

2. Which 1997 film, directed by James Cameron, became the highest-grossing film of all time until the 2000s?
   a. Jurassic Park
   b. Titanic
   c. The Matrix

d. Star Wars: Episode I – The Phantom Menace

3. What was the name of the first successfully cloned mammal in 1996, a sheep?
   a. Dolly
   b. Molly
   c. Polly
   d. Holly

4. Which popular TV sitcom, running from 1994 to 2004, followed the lives of six friends living in New York City?
   a. Friends
   b. Seinfeld
   c. Frasier
   d. The Fresh Prince of Bel-Air

5. In 1991, which country dissolved, leading to the independence of its constituent republics?
   a. Soviet Union
   b. Yugoslavia
   c. Czechoslovakia
   d. East Germany

6. Who became the world's richest person in 1995, thanks to his technology company?
   a. Bill Gates
   b. Warren Buffett
   c. Steve Jobs
   d. Jeff Bezos

7. Which musical artist, known as the "King of Pop," faced allegations of child molestation in the 1990s?
   a. Michael Jackson

    b. Prince

    c. Madonna

    d. Whitney Houston

8. In 1992, which city hosted the Summer Olympics, known for the debut of the Dream Team in basketball?

    a. Atlanta

    b. Barcelona

    c. Sydney

    d. Seoul

9. Which video game console, released in 1994, became a significant rival to Nintendo and Sega in the console wars?

    a. Sony PlayStation

    b. Microsoft Xbox

    c. Nintendo 64

    d. Sega Saturn

10. What was the name of the peace agreement signed in 1995 that brought an end to the Bosnian War?

    a. The Dayton Accords

    b. The Paris Peace Agreement

    c. The Oslo Accords

    d. The Treaty of Versailles

11. Which treaty, signed in 1993, created a free trade zone between the United States, Canada, and Mexico?

    a. The North American Free Trade Agreement (NAFTA)

    b. The Trans-Pacific Partnership (TPP)

    c. The European Union (EU)

    d. The Central American Free Trade Agreement (CAFTA)

12. In 1995, a federal building in which U.S. city was bombed, resulting

in significant loss of life?

   a. Oklahoma City

   b. New York City

   c. Los Angeles

   d. Chicago

13. Which company launched Windows 95, a major advancement in personal computing, in 1995?

   a. Apple

   b. IBM

   c. Microsoft

   d. Sun Microsystems

14. Who was the lead singer of the band Nirvana, which became a symbol of the grunge movement of the early 90s?

   a. Eddie Vedder

   b. Kurt Cobain

   c. Chris Cornell

   d. Layne Staley

15. In 1990, Nelson Mandela was released from prison after 27 years. In which country did this occur?

   a. South Africa

   b. Kenya

   c. Nigeria

   d. Zimbabwe

16. Which landmark Internet browser was released by Netscape Communications in 1994?

   a. Internet Explorer

   b. Netscape Navigator

   c. Mozilla Firefox

   d. Opera

17. Which country won the 1994 FIFA World Cup, the first to be held in the United States?

   a. Brazil

   b. Italy

   c. Germany

   d. Argentina

18. Which animated Disney film, released in 1994, tells the story of a young lion cub's journey to adulthood and acceptance of his royal destiny?

   a. The Lion King

   b. Aladdin

   c. Beauty and the Beast

   d. Pocahontas

19. In 1992, the Maastricht Treaty was signed, formally establishing which political and economic union?

   a. The United Nations

   b. The Commonwealth of Nations

   c. The European Union

   d. The North Atlantic Treaty Organization

20. What was the name of the scandal involving President Bill Clinton and White House intern Monica Lewinsky?

   a. Watergate scandal

   b. Whitewater scandal

   c. Iran-Contra affair

   d. Lewinsky scandal

21. Which popular TV series, debuting in 1990, was known for its surreal and quirky narrative set in a small town?

   a. Twin Peaks

   b. The X-Files

c. Buffy the Vampire Slayer

d. Dawson's Creek

22. Who wrote 'Harry Potter and the Philosopher's Stone,' the first book in the Harry Potter series, published in 1997?

a. J.K. Rowling

b. Stephenie Meyer

c. Suzanne Collins

d. Philip Pullman

23. Which technology company went public in 1992 and became synonymous with the tech boom of the 90s?

a. Apple

b. Microsoft

c. IBM

d. Netscape

24. In 1991, which band released the album 'Nevermind,' which became a defining record of the grunge movement?

a. Nirvana

b. Pearl Jam

c. Soundgarden

d. Alice in Chains

25. Which international agreement aimed at reducing greenhouse gas emissions to combat global warming was adopted in 1997?

a. The Paris Agreement

b. The Kyoto Protocol

c. The Copenhagen Accord

d. The Montreal Protocol

26. What was the name of the sheep cloned in 1996, marking a significant breakthrough in biotechnology?

a. Dolly

b. Molly

c. Polly

d. Sally

27. Which iconic sitcom starring Jerry Seinfeld aired its final episode in 1998 to a record-breaking audience?

a. Friends

b. Seinfeld

c. Frasier

d. Cheers

28. Who was the female tennis player that dominated the sport throughout much of the 1990s?

a. Martina Navratilova

b. Monica Seles

c. Steffi Graf

d. Serena Williams

29. In 1991, which military operation was launched by the United States against Iraq in response to Iraq's invasion of Kuwait?

a. Operation Desert Storm

b. Operation Iraqi Freedom

c. Operation Enduring Freedom

d. Operation Anaconda

30. What was the popular dance craze of the early 1990s, featuring a song by Los Del Rio?

a. The Macarena

b. The Electric Slide

c. The Cha-Cha Slide

d. The Cupid Shuffle

31. Which popular children's show featuring a purple dinosaur debuted in 1992?
   a. Barney & Friends
   b. Teletubbies
   c. Blue's Clues
   d. Arthur

32. In 1995, which city in Japan was struck by a devastating earthquake, one of the deadliest in the country's history?
   a. Tokyo
   b. Kyoto
   c. Osaka
   d. Kobe

33. Which 1996 film starring Tom Cruise is known for its famous line, "You can't handle the truth!"?
   a. A Few Good Men
   b. Jerry Maguire
   c. Top Gun
   d. Mission: Impossible

34. In 1990, which country reunited after being divided post-World War II?
   a. Vietnam
   b. Germany
   c. Korea
   d. Yemen

35. What is the name of the telescope launched into space in 1990, providing new insights into the universe?
   a. James Webb Space Telescope
   b. Hubble Space Telescope
   c. Chandra X-ray Observatory

d. Spitzer Space Telescope

36. Who was the famous rapper and actor who starred in the sitcom 'The Fresh Prince of Bel-Air,' which began in 1990?

a. Ice Cube
b. LL Cool J
c. Tupac Shakur
d. Will Smith

37. In 1992, which hurricane caused significant damage in Florida, becoming one of the most destructive in U.S. history?

a. Hurricane Andrew
b. Hurricane Katrina
c. Hurricane Sandy
d. Hurricane Irma

38. Which 1999 movie, directed by the Wachowskis, is known for its innovative visual effects and exploration of virtual reality?

a. The Matrix
b. Blade Runner
c. Inception
d. Total Recall

39. In 1994, which figure skater was attacked in a scandal that led to one of the biggest controversies in sports history?

a. Nancy Kerrigan
b. Tonya Harding
c. Michelle Kwan
d. Kristi Yamaguchi

40. What was the popular animated TV show that debuted in 1997, known for its satirical humor and adult themes?

a. Family Guy

b. South Park

c. The Simpsons

d. Futurama

One Special Memory from the 90s

"The Launch of the Hubble Space Telescope - In 1990, this telescope was launched into space, providing humanity with unprecedented views of the universe and revolutionizing our understanding of the cosmos."

As we conclude our nostalgic journey through the 1990s, let's appreciate how this trip down memory lane has revisited key moments that shaped the close of the twentieth century.

The next section lists all the answers to our trivia questions, offering you a chance to reflect on how well you remember these dynamic decades.

7

ANSWERS

Answers Chapter 1: The Fifties

1. Answer: a. Harry S. Truman
2. Answer: a. Cinderella
3. Answer: b. China
4. Answer: b. Rock 'n' Roll
5. Answer: b. Sputnik 1
6. Answer: a. George Orwell
7. Answer: b. 4 minutes
8. Answer: c. The Wild One
9. Answer: c. 1955
10. Answer: c. Cuba
11. Answer: b. Buddy Holly
12. Answer: a. Lucille Ball
13. Answer: d. Bonanza
14. Answer: b. J.D. Salinger
15. Answer: b. Brown v. Board of Education
16. Answer: b. Scrabble
17. Answer: b. Rock 'n' Roll

18. Answer: a. Queen Elizabeth II
19. Answer: a. Polio
20. Answer: c. Marilyn Monroe
21. Answer: a. "Nice lady!"
22. Answer: c. Jackie Robinson
23. Answer: a. Vladimir Nabokov
24. Answer: b. Chevrolet Bel Air
25. Answer: b. The first artificial satellite, Sputnik, was launched.
26. Answer: b. Slinky
27. Answer: c. Rear Window
28. Answer: b. Russia
29. Answer: c. West Side Story
30. Answer: b. Elvis Presley
31. Answer: b. I Love Lucy
32. Answer: c. De Havilland Comet
33. Answer: b. London
34. Answer: c. Ray Bradbury
35. Answer: b. 12 Angry Men
36. Answer: d. Rock 'n' Roll
37. Answer: b. Vietnam
38. Answer: a. The Twilight Zone
39. Answer: a. Ernest Hemingway
40. Answer: a. The Suez Crisis

Answers Chapter 2: The Sixties

1. Answer: a. Neil Armstrong
2. Answer: a. The Beatles
3. Answer: b. Martin Luther King Jr.
4. Answer: b. The Graduate

5. Answer: b. The Cuban Missile Crisis

6. Answer: b. Woodstock

7. Answer: a. Lee Harvey Oswald

8. Answer: a. To Kill a Mockingbird

9. Answer: c. Alan Shepard

10. Answer: b. The Minibus

11. Answer: c. 24th Amendment

12. Answer: b. Harold Wilson

13. Answer: d. I Spy

14. Answer: d. All of the above

15. Answer: a. Joseph Heller

16. Answer: a. The birth control pill

17. Answer: c. Butch Cassidy and the Sundance Kid

18. Answer: b. The Congo

19. Answer: c. A landslide

20. Answer: b. Thurgood Marshall

21. Answer: b. Gilligan's Island

22. Answer: a. Pet Sounds

23. Answer: b. The March on Washington

24. Answer: c. 1964

25. Answer: b. Psycho

26. Answer: b. Martin Luther King Jr.

27. Answer: a. Ford Mustang

28. Answer: b. Valentina Tereshkova

29. Answer: c. 2001: A Space Odyssey

30. Answer: b. 23rd Amendment

31. Answer: a. The Beatles

32. Answer: c. Operation Rolling Thunder

33. Answer: b. Silent Spring

34. Answer: a. Muhammad Ali

35. Answer: b. West Side Story

36. Answer: c. Ghana

37. Answer: c. The Manson Family murders

38. Answer: c. Richard Nixon
39. Answer: a. The publication of "The Feminine Mystique"
40. Answer: b. The Human Be-In

Answers Chapter 3: The Seventies

1. Answer: a. Richard Nixon
2. Answer: b. Jaws
3. Answer: c. The Hustle
4. Answer: b. The Walkman
5. Answer: c. Margaret Thatcher
6. Answer: a. 1973
7. Answer: a. Star Wars: A New Hope
8. Answer: c. Skylab
9. Answer: b. Punk Rock
10. Answer: a. Bangladesh
11. Answer: b. Earth Day
12. Answer: a. Space Invaders
13. Answer: a. Richard Nixon
14. Answer: b. Ted Bundy
15. Answer: a. Elvis Presley
16. Answer: c. Watergate Scandal
17. Answer: b. Roe v. Wade
18. Answer: b. Muhammad Ali
19. Answer: a. Rocky
20. Answer: b. Netherlands
21. Answer: a. The Beatles
22. Answer: c. Volkswagen
23. Answer: a. Clean Air Act
24. Answer: b. Ronald Wayne

25. Answer: a. MASH
26. Answer: b. The Dark Side of the Moon
27. Answer: a. Madeleine Albright
28. Answer: c. The Iranian Revolution
29. Answer: a. Three Mile Island
30. Answer: a. Space Invaders
31. Answer: b. The Camp David Accords
32. Answer: b. Paul Allen
33. Answer: b. A Clockwork Orange
34. Answer: a. Switzerland
35. Answer: a. Bruce Lee
36. Answer: a. Woodstock
37. Answer: c. William Friedkin
38. Answer: a. Atari 2600
39. Answer: b. Regents of the University of California v. Bakke
40. Answer: a. "Imagine"

Answers Chapter 4: The Eighties

1. Answer: a. Ronald Reagan
2. Answer: c. Back to the Future
3. Answer: c. Chernobyl
4. Answer: a. Michael Jackson
5. Answer: c. VCR
6. Answer: a. Challenger
7. Answer: a. Margaret Thatcher
8. Answer: b. Super Mario Bros.
9. Answer: b. Sandra Day O'Connor
10. Answer: c. HIV/AIDS
11. Answer: b. Seinfeld

12. Answer: c. "Video Killed the Radio Star" by The Buggles
13. Answer: c. Back to the Future
14. Answer: a. Aretha Franklin
15. Answer: c. Travel into space
16. Answer: a. Die Hard
17. Answer: b. Nintendo Entertainment System
18. Answer: b. Soviet Union
19. Answer: a. Miami Vice
20. Answer: b. Exxon Valdez oil spill
21. Answer: c. Aerobics
22. Answer: a. The Handmaid's Tale
23. Answer: b. Omnibot
24. Answer: b. Michael Jackson
25. Answer: a. Top Gun
26. Answer: b. Live Aid
27. Answer: d. Luxo Jr.
28. Answer: d. Bjorn Borg
29. Answer: a. United States
30. Answer: b. Thriller
31. Answer: b. Mikhail Gorbachev
32. Answer: b. John Rambo
33. Answer: c. V
34. Answer: c. Pac-Man
35. Answer: a. The Bonfire of the Vanities
36. Answer: a. Vincent van Gogh
37. Answer: b. Bhopal gas tragedy
38. Answer: c. Tim Berners-Lee
39. Answer: a. Stephen King
40. Answer: c. Vanessa Williams

Answers Chapter 5: The Nineties

1. Answer: b. Bill Clinton
2. Answer: b. Titanic
3. Answer: a. Dolly
4. Answer: a. Friends
5. Answer: a. Soviet Union
6. Answer: a. Bill Gates
7. Answer: a. Michael Jackson
8. Answer: b. Barcelona
9. Answer: a. Sony PlayStation
10. Answer: a. The Dayton Accords
11. Answer: a. The North American Free Trade Agreement (NAFTA)
12. Answer: a. Oklahoma City
13. Answer: c. Microsoft
14. Answer: b. Kurt Cobain
15. Answer: a. South Africa
16. Answer: b. Netscape Navigator
17. Answer: a. Brazil
18. Answer: a. The Lion King
19. Answer: c. The European Union
20. Answer: d. Lewinsky scandal
21. Answer: a. Twin Peaks
22. Answer: a. J.K. Rowling
23. Answer: d. Netscape
24. Answer: a. Nirvana
25. Answer: b. The Kyoto Protocol
26. Answer: a. Dolly
27. Answer: b. Seinfeld
28. Answer: c. Steffi Graf
29. Answer: a. Operation Desert Storm
30. Answer: a. The Macarena

31. Answer: a. Barney & Friends
32. Answer: d. Kobe
33. Answer: a. A Few Good Men
34. Answer: b. Germany
35. Answer: b. Hubble Space Telescope
36. Answer: d. Will Smith
37. Answer: a. Hurricane Andrew
38. Answer: a. The Matrix
39. Answer: a. Nancy Kerrigan
40. Answer: b. South Park

8

CONCLUSION

As we conclude our journey through the vibrant eras from the Fifties to the Nineties, it's clear that each decade has left a unique imprint on our collective memory.

Through this "Trivia For Seniors" book, we aimed to not just entertain but also to engage and educate.

It has been a delightful journey, piecing together the puzzles of the past, rediscovering the charm of yesteryears, and perhaps, learning something new along the way. This book serves as a bridge connecting the past and the present, offering a chance to reflect on how far we have come and the remarkable events that have led us here.

As we turn the final page, I hope that this book has brought joy, sparked conversation, and rekindled fond memories. Whether you journeyed through these pages alone or shared the experience with friends and family, it's been an honor to accompany you on this nostalgic expedition.

If you've enjoyed this trip through the decades, I invite you to leave a review on Amazon. Your feedback not only helps us but also guides fellow readers in their quest for engaging and enriching reads. Please share your thoughts, favorite moments, and how this book has touched your journey down memory lane.

Thank you for choosing to relive history with us. May the memories and stories enclosed in these pages continue to inspire and bring joy to you and those around you.

9

REFERENCES

Historical events and figures: History.com

Information on movies and TV shows: IMDb (Internet Movie Database)

Sports-related trivia, especially baseball: Baseball-Reference.com

Biographies of famous personalities from the 1950s: Biography.com

Space-related events and technological advancements: NASA.gov

Music and cultural events related to rock 'n' roll: Rockhall.com (Rock & Roll Hall of Fame)

OpenAI. (2024). *ChatGPT* (4) [Large language model]. https://chat.openai.com

About the Author

Virin Gomber (Mindful Solutions Publishing) is a Success Coach, Author, and Motivational Speaker. He has co-authored another popular Amazon book, "The Missing Piece in Self-Love: Love Yourself from the Inside Out."

Mindful Solutions Publishing is a distinguished brand specializing in the diverse fields of Health, Fitness, Well-being, Self-Help, Psychology, Relationships, Communication, Life Success, and more, offering an array of insightful and transformative books.

At Mindful Solutions Publishing, we recognize the unique journey of each individual seeking to improve their health and personal wellness. Our collection of books is meticulously curated to address a variety of needs, from beginners seeking foundational knowledge to those delving into more advanced practices for physical and emotional well-being.

Embark on a Nostalgic Journey Through Time with "Trivia for Seniors."

"Trivia for Seniors" is crafted to intrigue minds of all backgrounds with a rich tapestry of topics, ensuring there's something for everyone.